More Fruits and Vegetables Travel to Mr. Heart 2

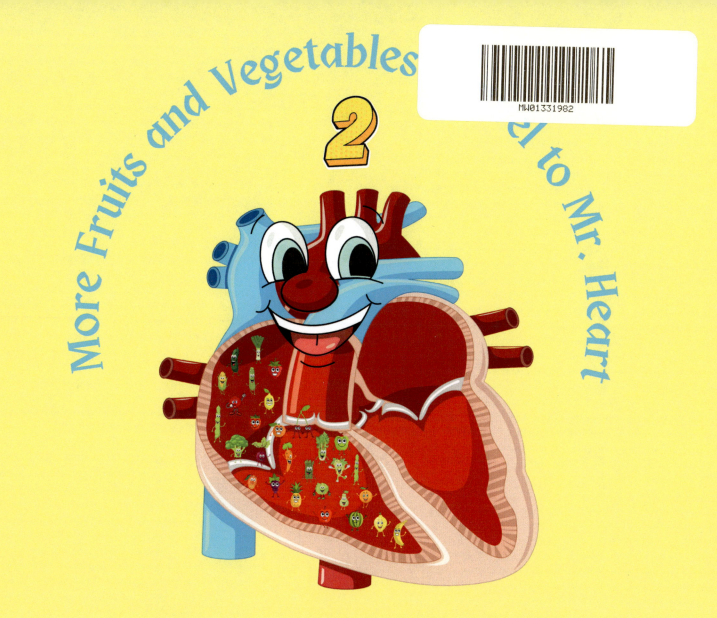

Pat Broadney

Illustrated by Sangi Parvin

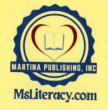

MARTINA PUBLISHING, INC
MsLiteracy.com

Text copyright ©2024 Patricia Broadney. All rights reserved under International Copyright Law. No part of this book may be reproduced in any form or by any means without the author's prior written consent.

Martina Publishing, Inc.
www.MsLiteracy.com

More Fruits and Vegetables Travel to Mr. Heart
Written by Patricia Broadney. Illustrated by Sangi Parvin.

Summary:
This is the second book in the Travel to Mr. Heart series. Readers will discover the origins of fruits and vegetables, how they can be consumed, and the health benefits they bring to Mr. Heart. This book is perfect for both adults and children to read together as a means of promoting health.

[1. Fruits-Healthy Foods. 2. Vegetables-Healthy Foods. 3. Heart-Healthy Living. I. Title.]

ISBN: 9781957645193
Library of Congress Control Number: 2024922983

©2024 Printed in the United States of America

Dedication:

To those who desire to live healthy.

Acknowledgements:

I would like to acknowledge my Lord and Savior Jesus Christ, my husband Kenneth of 28 years, and my two protégés. Just to name a few others, Mrs. Williams, Mrs. Johnson, and my school bus driver encouraged me to go after my career.

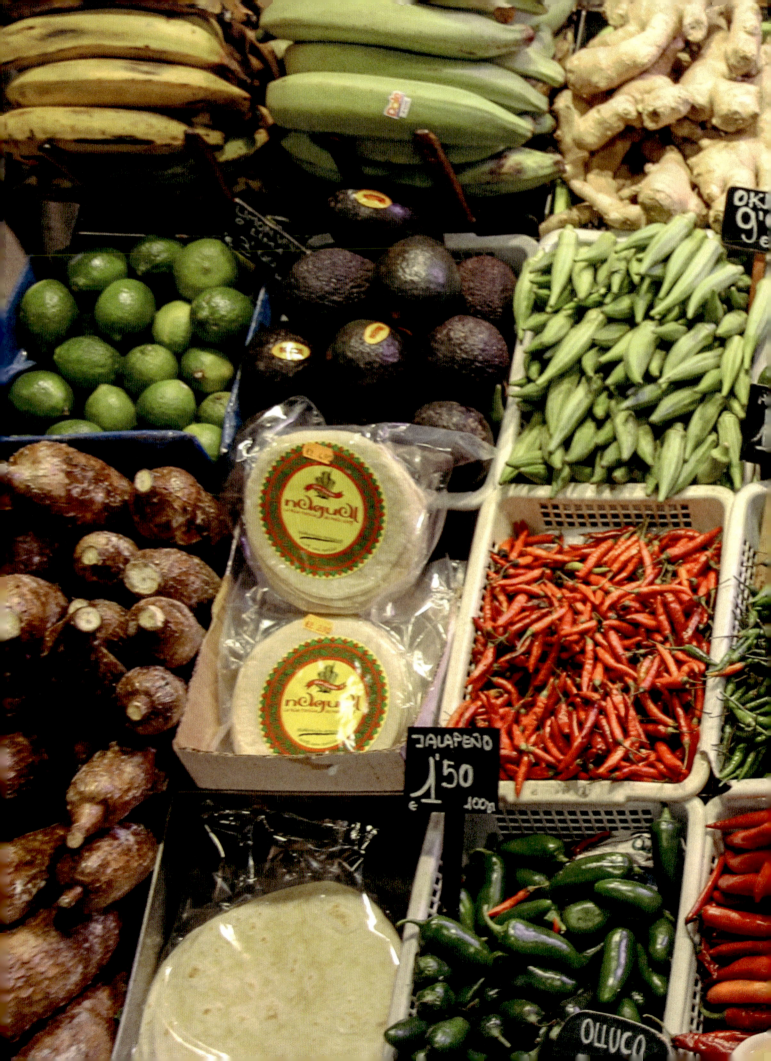

We now know that fruits and vegetables make the heart happy and healthy and that God nurtures them with rain and sunlight.

Most colorful fruits and vegetables have anti-inflammatory and antioxidant compounds. Let's explore more about fruits and vegetables we can enjoy as they nurture Mr. Heart.

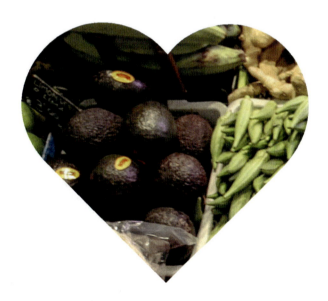

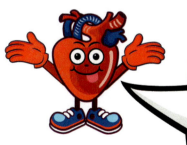

Red food gives you a strong heart. Orange food helps you see in the dark. Yellow food helps your body heal cuts. Green food helps you fight off sickness. Blue and purple foods give you a strong brain. White food gives you energy.

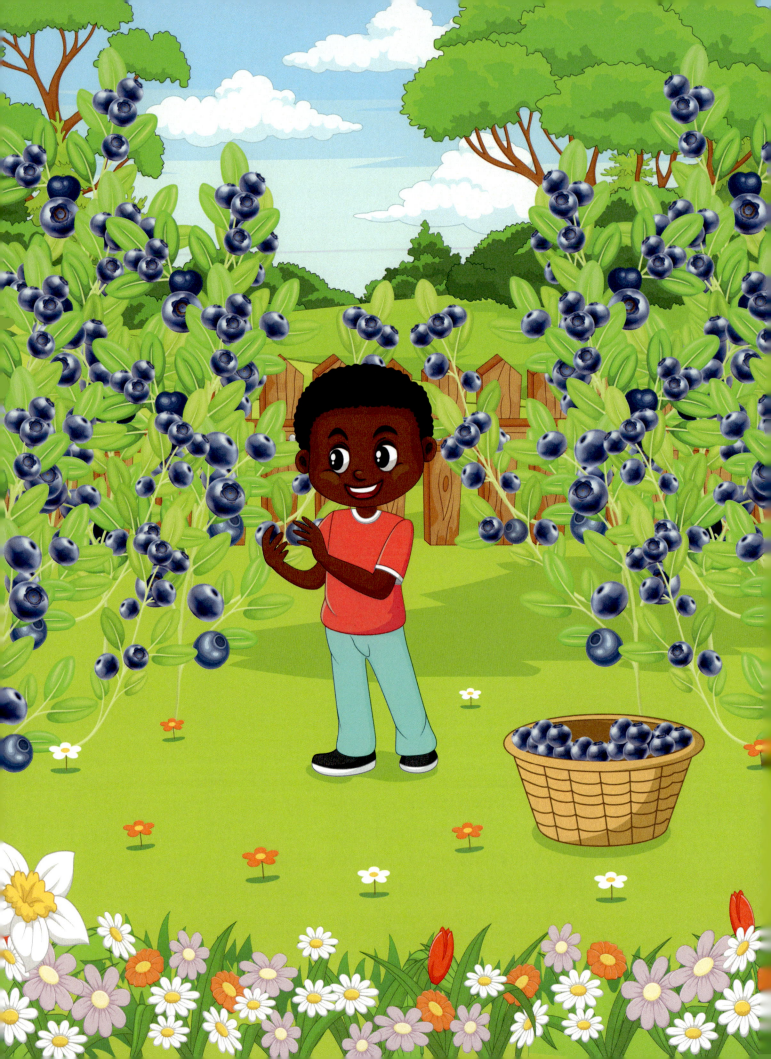

Tez picks blueberries in July during his trips to the berry fields known as barrens. He munches on these delicious, succulent fruits. Mmmm, good!

These berries help lower the bad cholesterol in your blood and kicks out the extra sugar in the bloodstream.

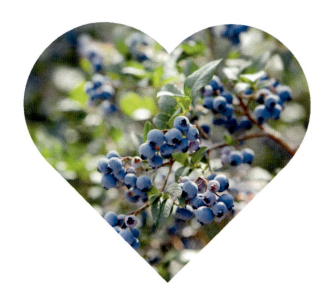

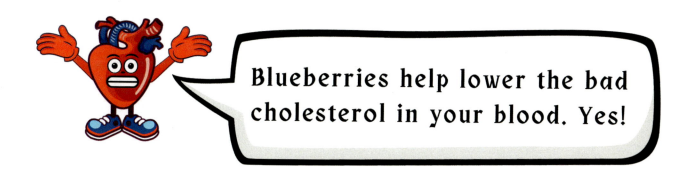

Blueberries help lower the bad cholesterol in your blood. Yes!

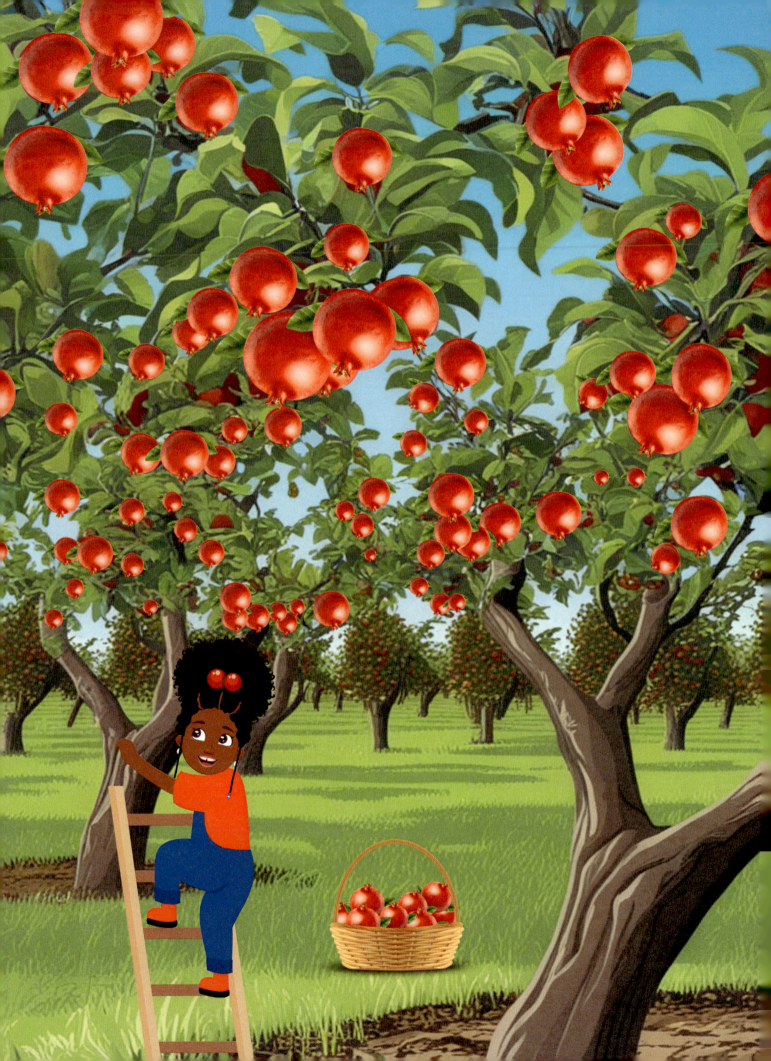

Lucy learns that there are 613 pomegranate seeds, the same as the 613 laws from the Old Testament in the Bible.

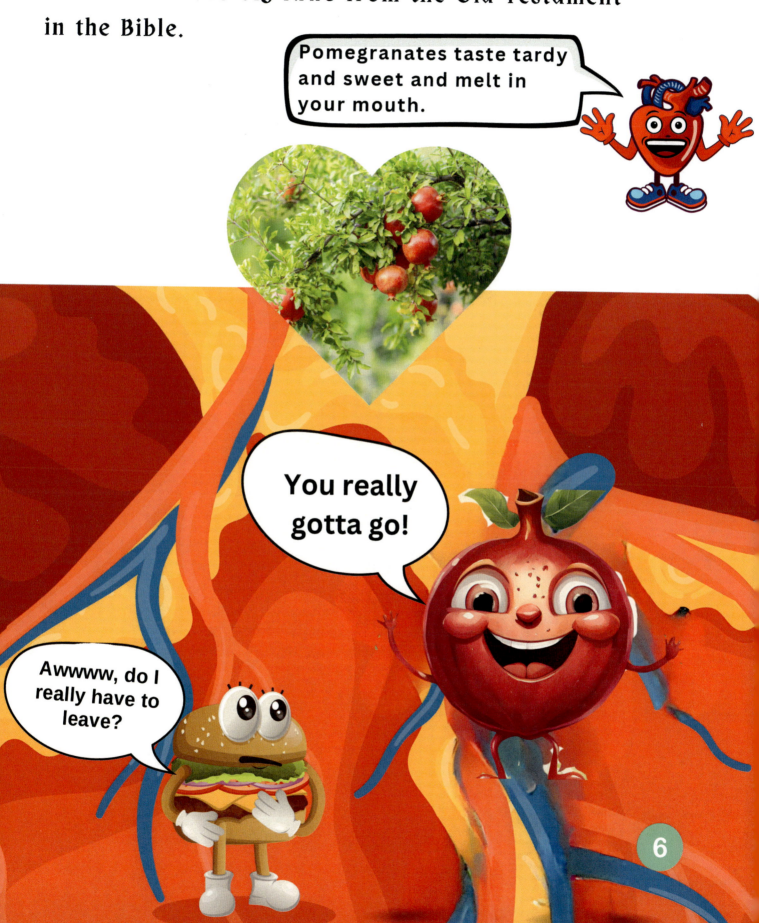

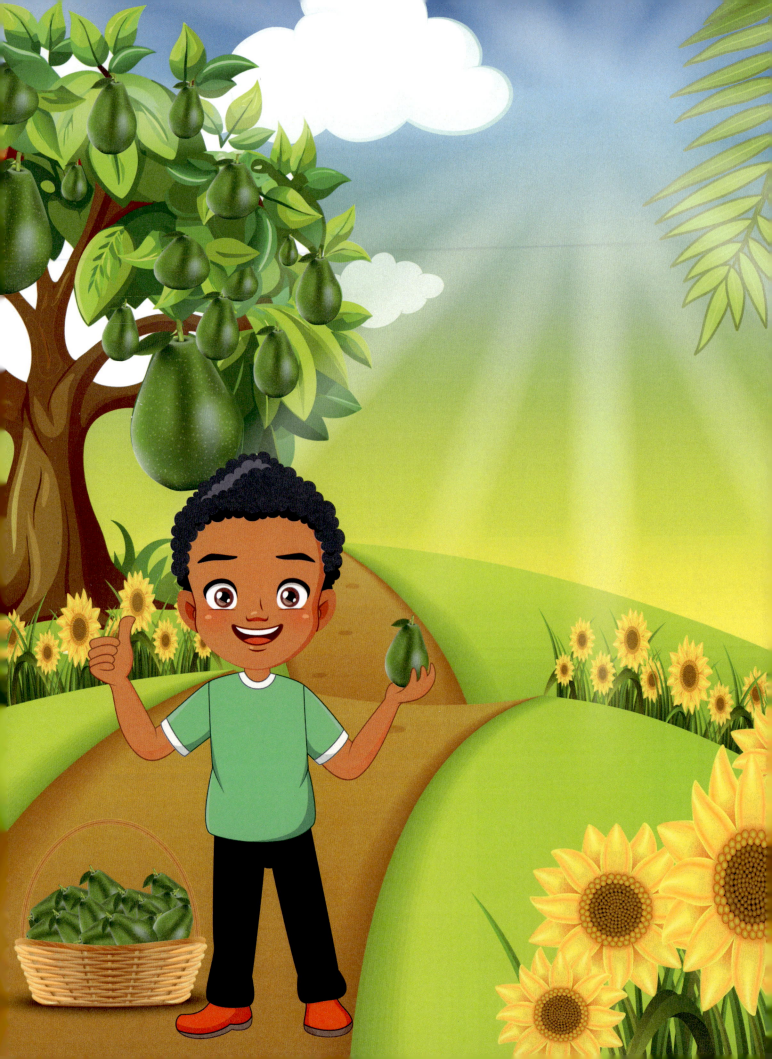

Roberto found out that avocados are fruits that grow on trees in Mexico and Central America. He learned how to cut the avocado by slicing through the skin. He pushes through until the knife hits the seed. After that, he twists it apart, revealing the firm, light green delicious flesh inside.

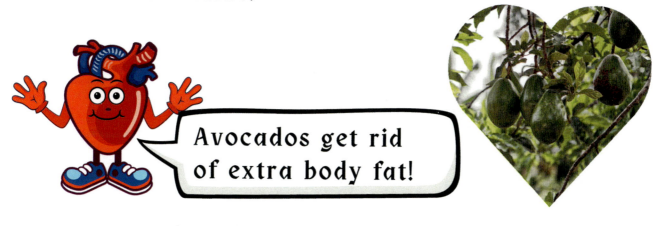

Avocados get rid of extra body fat!

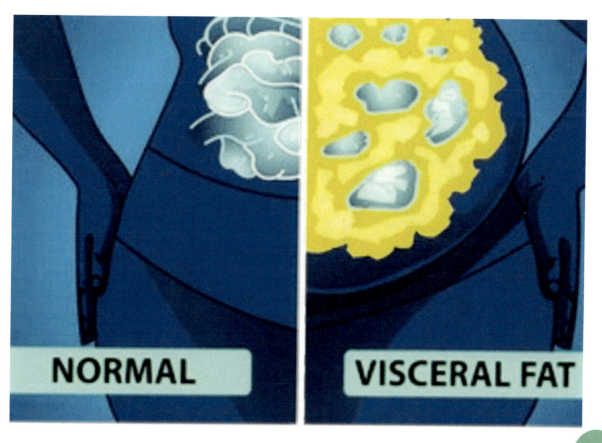

NORMAL VISCERAL FAT

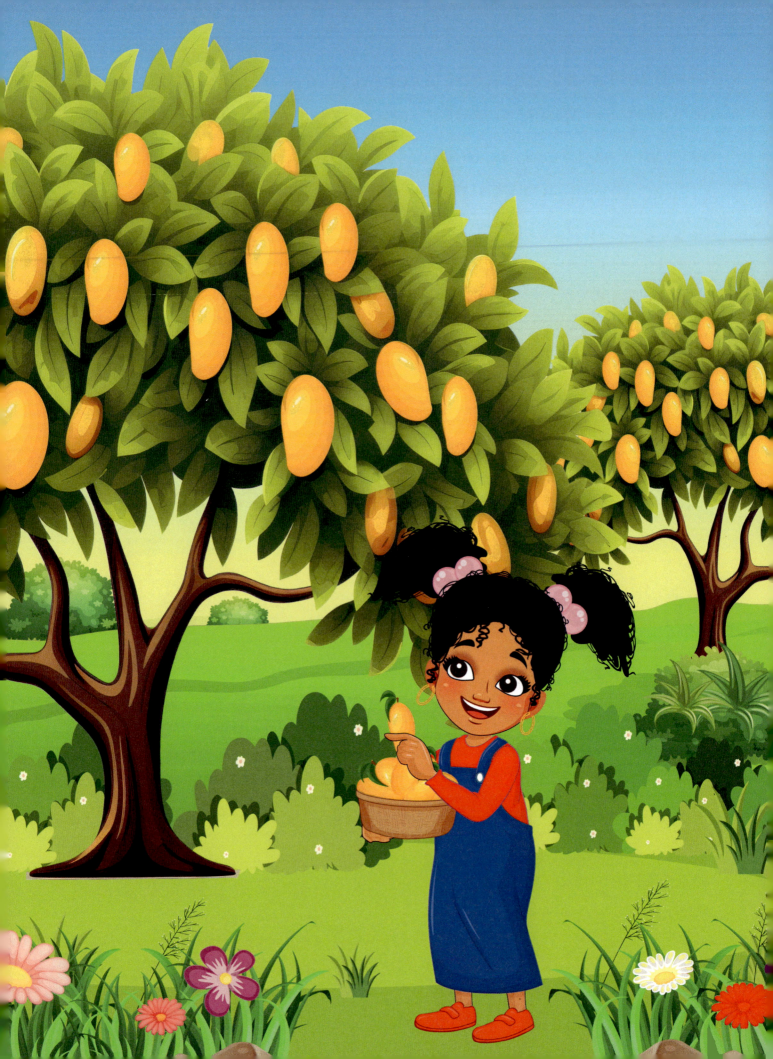

Sonya goes to the field to pick nice, firm mangoes from the tree. Mangoes are the perfect fruit for a delicious snack, and they are tasty and smooth.

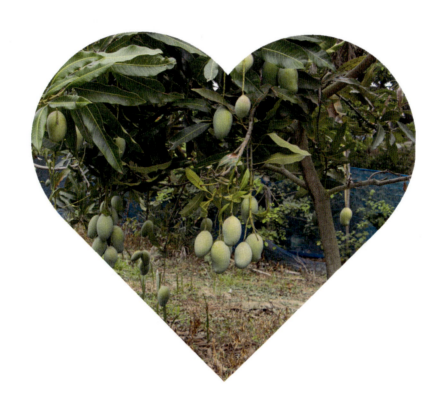

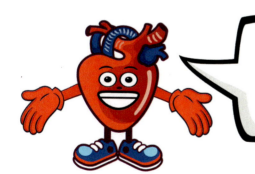

Mangoes provide a great source of magnesium, potassium, and antioxidants for a healthy body.

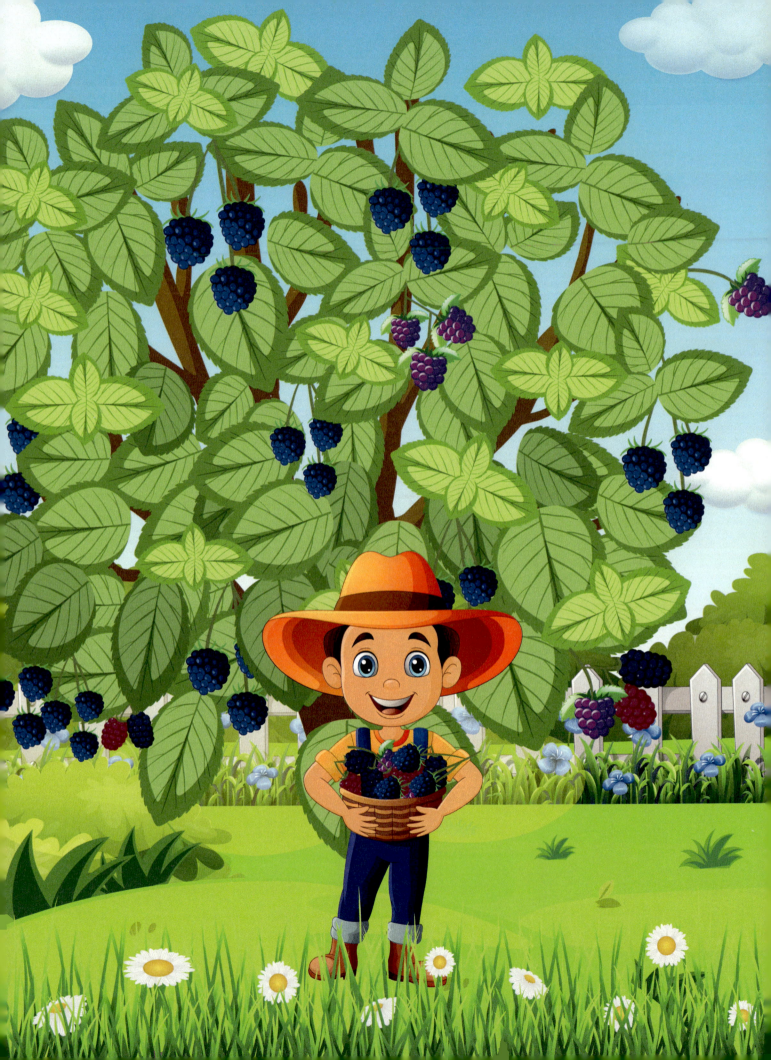

Kenneth loves to pick very dark purple blackberries from the edge of the backyards. He can't stay away from them because they are so delicious. The heart loves them because they bring nourishment to keep it pumping.

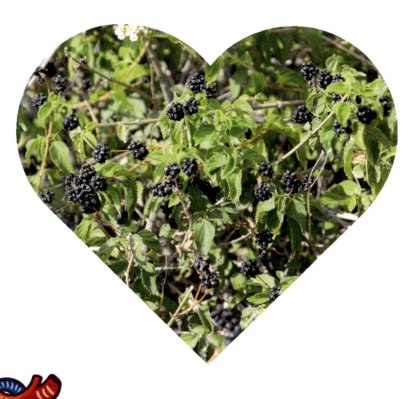

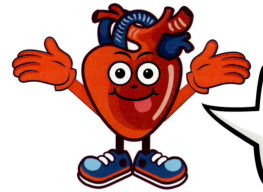

Blackberries are not true berries but fruit from woody plants. Blackberries are a superfood rich in Vitamins C, K, and manganese.

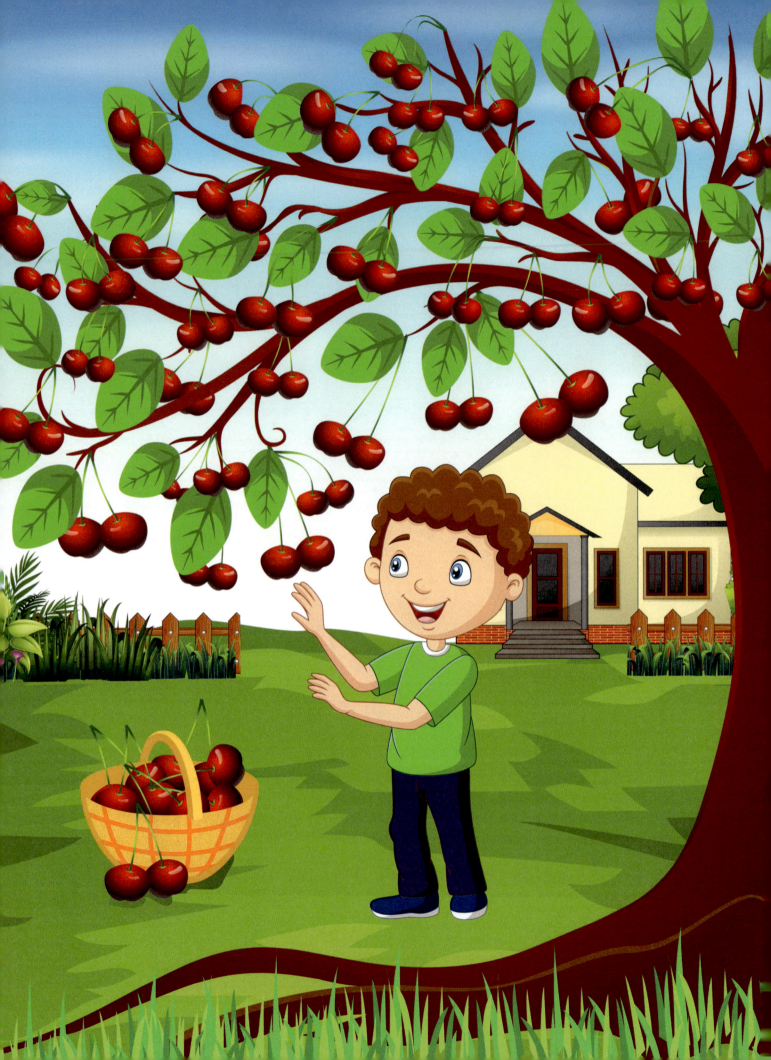

Carlos enjoys picking cherries from his papa's trees after they turn red. Sometimes, Carlos can't get to sleep at night, so he crunches and munches on a few cherries. Sometimes, his shoulders, elbows, knees, and toes hurt from picking so many cherries. Then, he remembers when Grandpa was hurting that Grandma gave him some delicious cherry juice to flush the irritating arthritis out of his body.

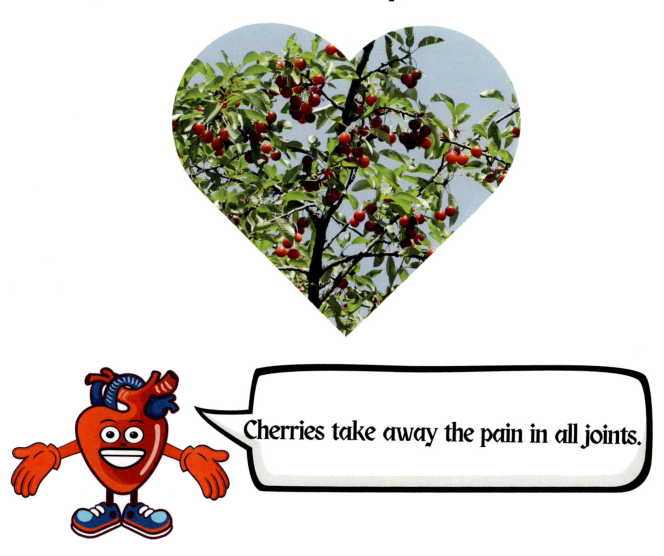

Cherries take away the pain in all joints.

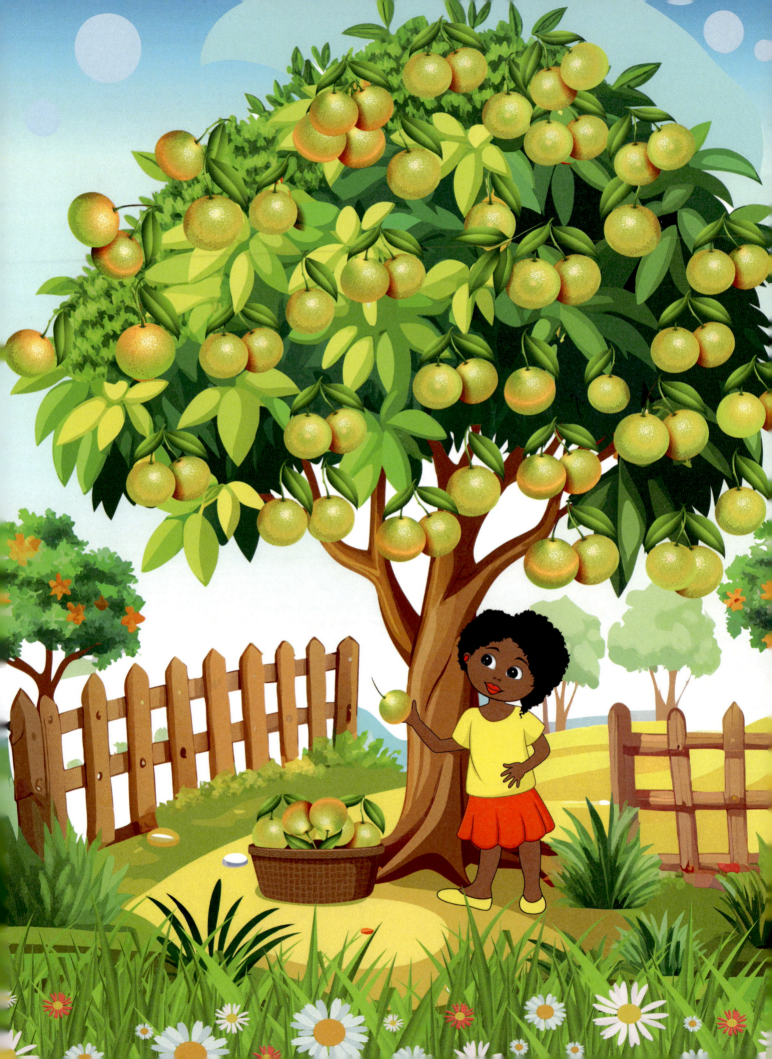

Karen studies oranges because she loves the sweet taste and soothing smell released after ripping the skin.

These oranges travel a long way to get to where we live, from Australia and South Africa. They are full of vitamins, like Vitamin C and folate. The smell of oranges makes your brain think happy thoughts and causes your heart to burst with excitement.

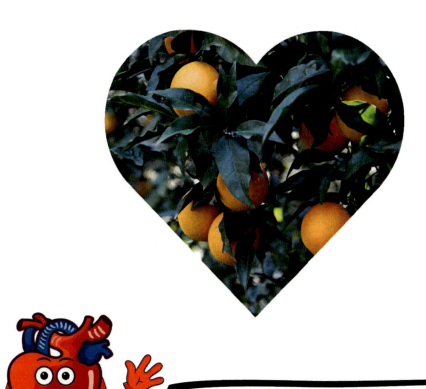

Oranges provide Vitamin and potassium. They support a healthy heart and prevent kidney stones.

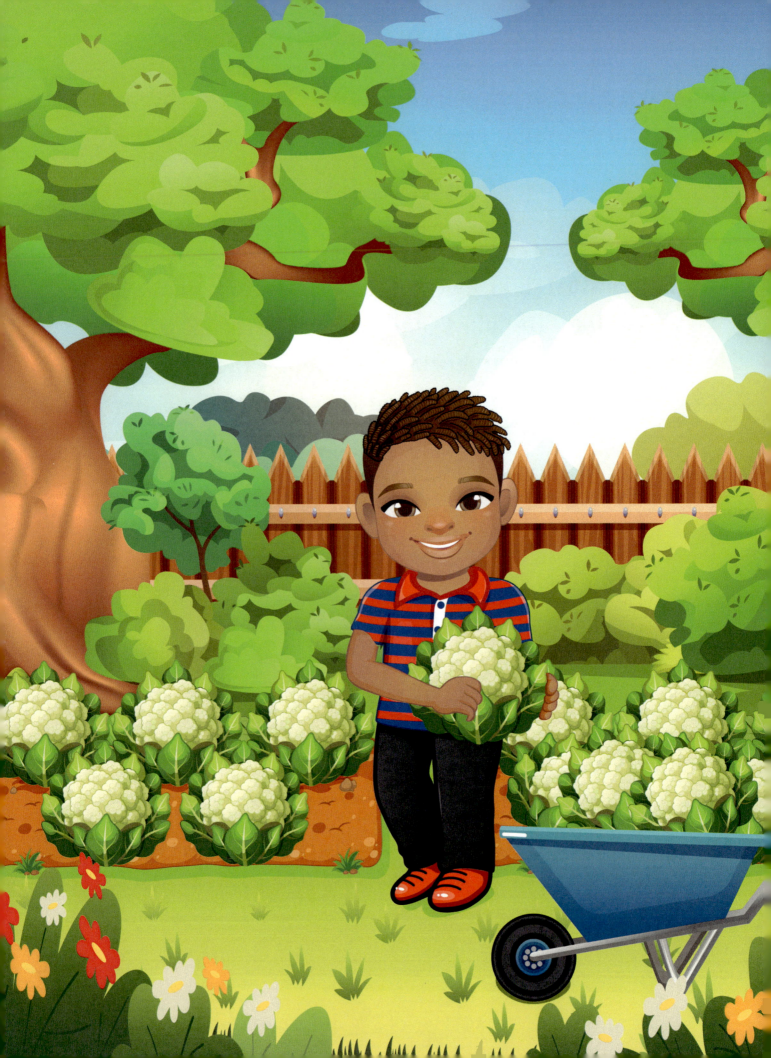

Pedro likes the look of a cauliflower because it reminds him of broccoli. Mmm, good.

The flesh of the cauliflower is sometimes called "curd." The Italian word "cavolifiore" means "cabbage flower." This vegetable slows the aging process, protects your brain against disease, and helps you think better.

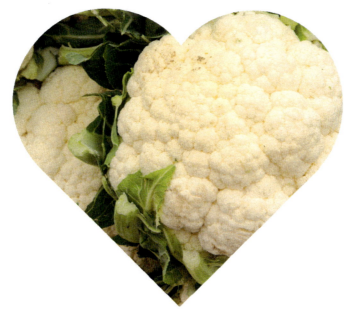

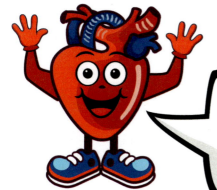

Cauliflower is a superfood because it stops cancer cells from growing.

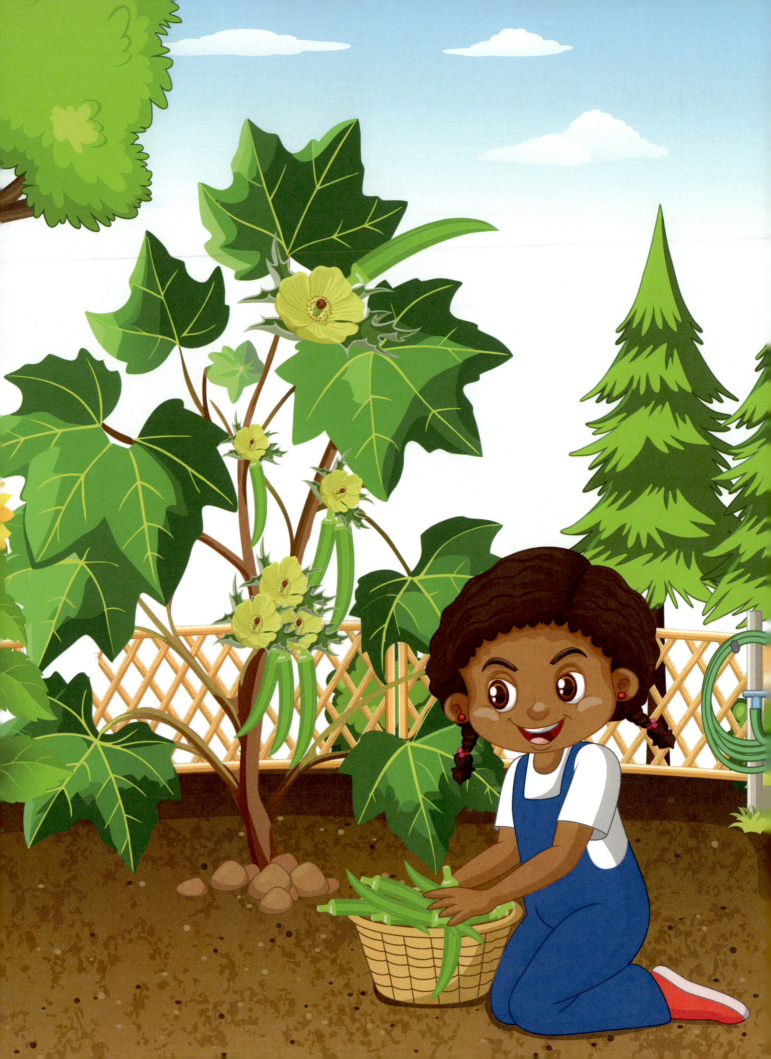

Kaylie uses the "slime" of okra to help her stomach ache calm down. She goes out early in the morning to pick those green, pointy okra from her farm in Georgia.

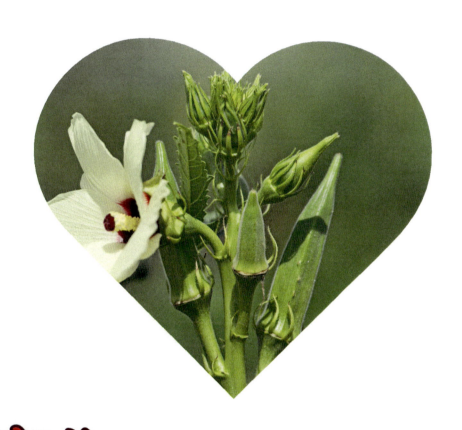

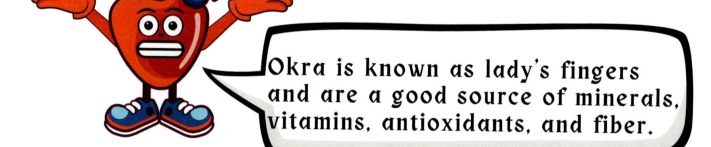

Okra is known as lady's fingers and are a good source of minerals, vitamins, antioxidants, and fiber.

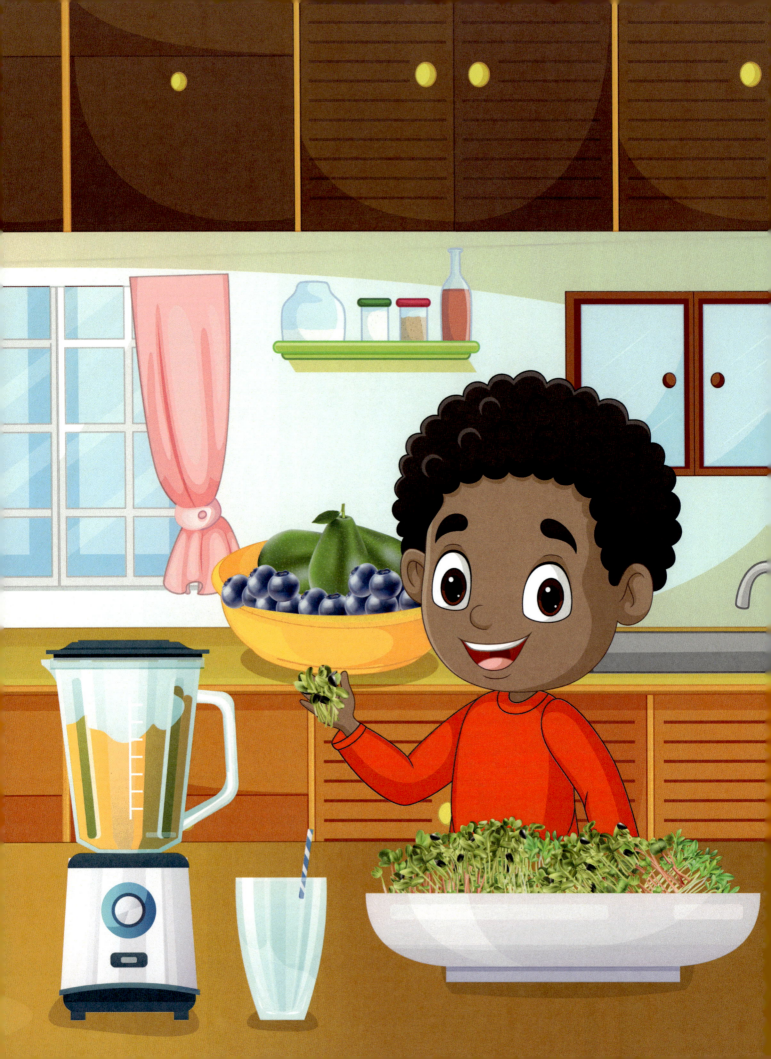

Michael throws Microgreens into the blender to make an energy soup instead of a salad. They are small veggies cut just after leaves appear on a stem. They are power-packed small plants that nourish us with Vitamins C, E, K, and A. We need them for our bones to grow strong and healthy.

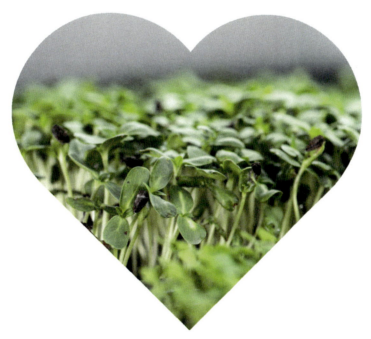

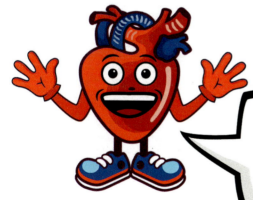

Add avocado, pineapple, sunflower seeds, chia seeds, juice, and water for a great smoothie.

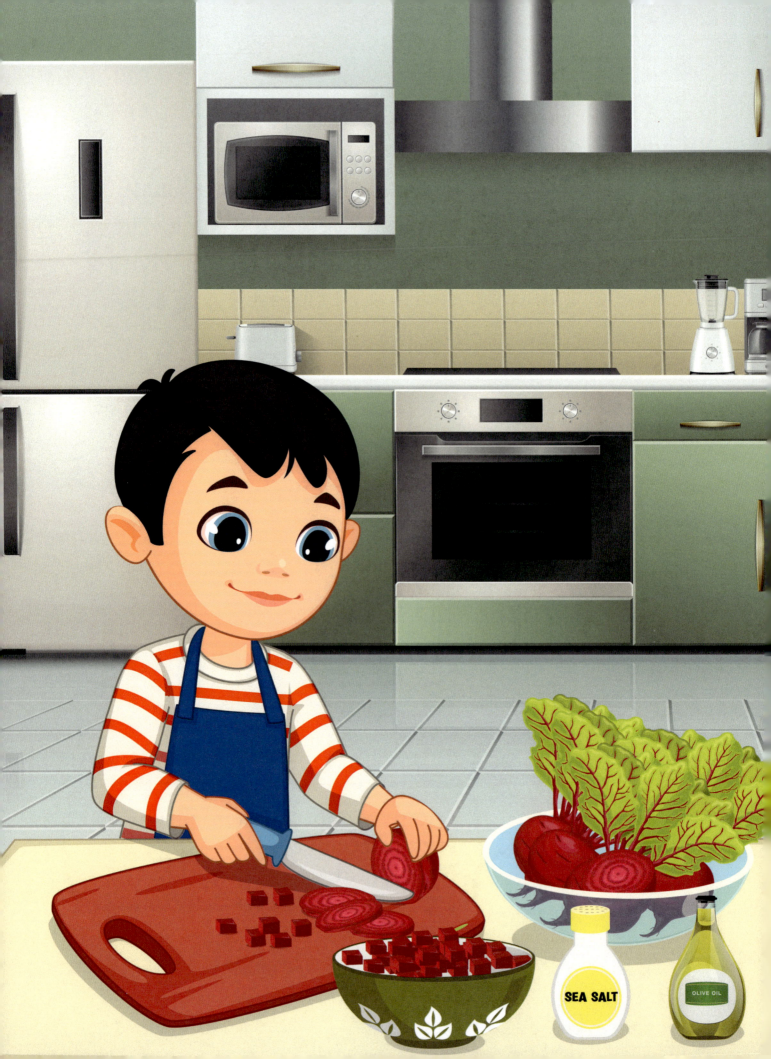

Burt loves to snack on beets, cut into small chunks, baked with olive oil, and seasoned with a pinch of sea salt after being baked in the oven.

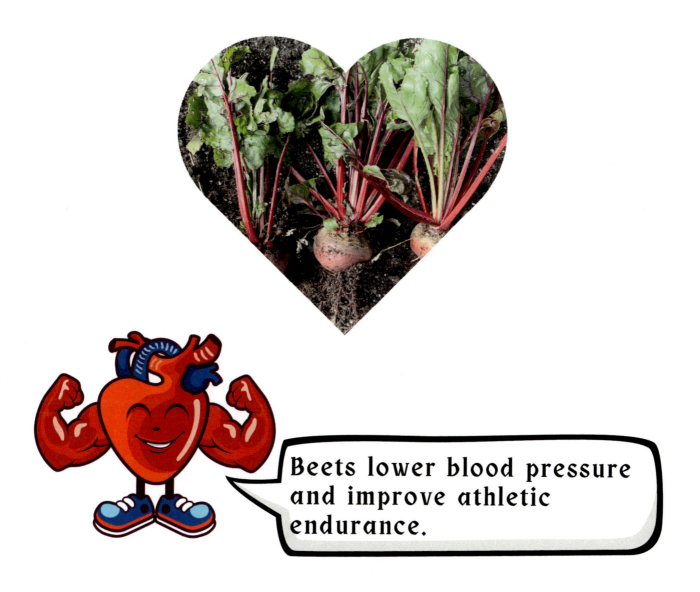

Beets lower blood pressure and improve athletic endurance.

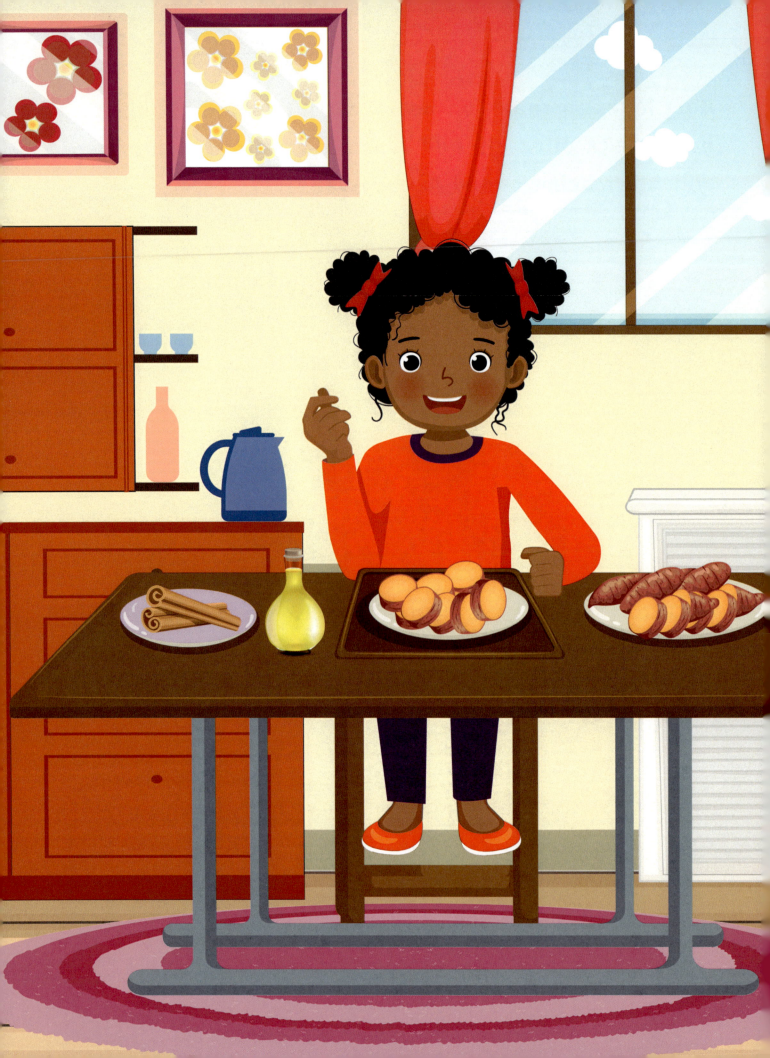

Sasha can't stop eating those sweet potatoes drizzled with olive oil with just a tad bit of cinnamon. Between you and me, they replenish our bodies with antioxidants and keep swelling down throughout our bodies. When the sun wants to damage our skin, those sweet potatoes protect our skin from the bad things in our environment.

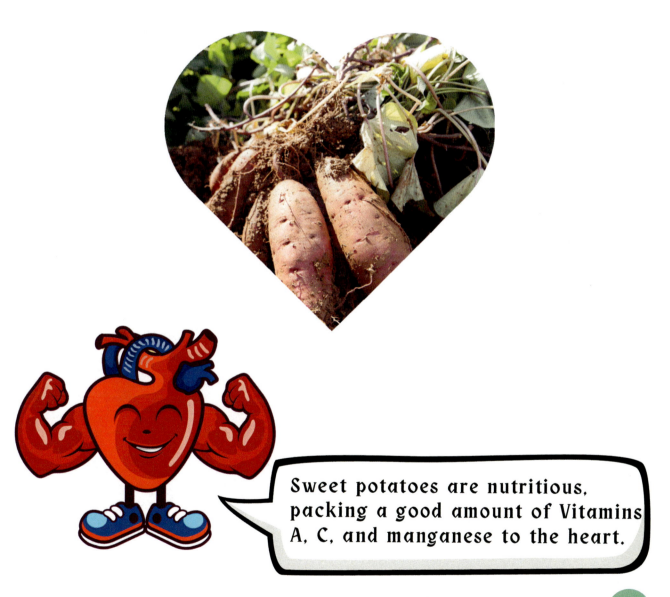

Sweet potatoes are nutritious, packing a good amount of Vitamins A, C, and manganese to the heart.

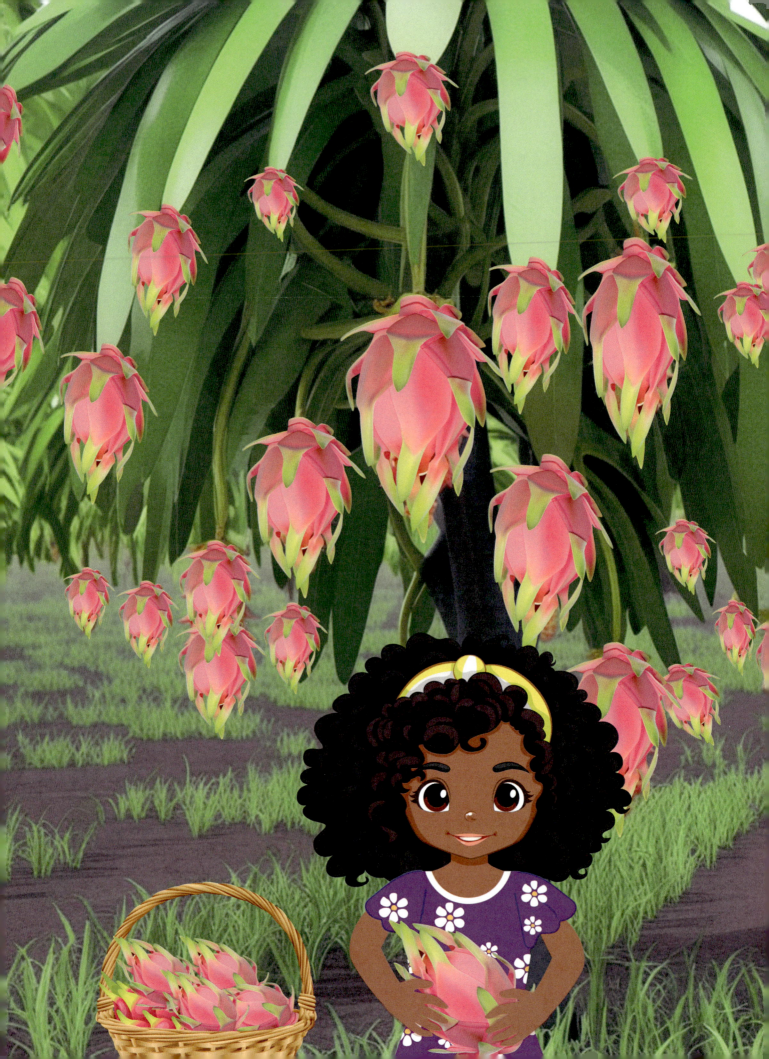

Takerria slices the soft purple skin of the Dragon fruit, revealing the white sweet speckled pulp. She receives all the nutrients from the fruit, such as Vitamins C and E. It's filled with nutrients like magnesium which helps to keep you calm. Prebiotics, help good bacteria grow, which means good digestion.

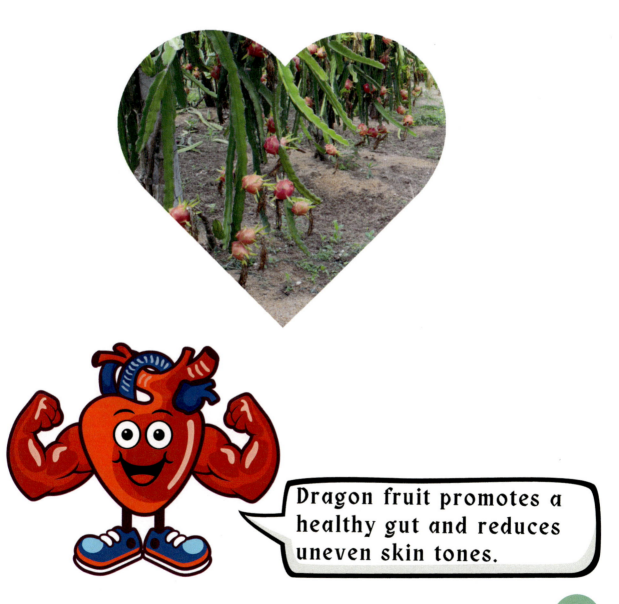

Dragon fruit promotes a healthy gut and reduces uneven skin tones.

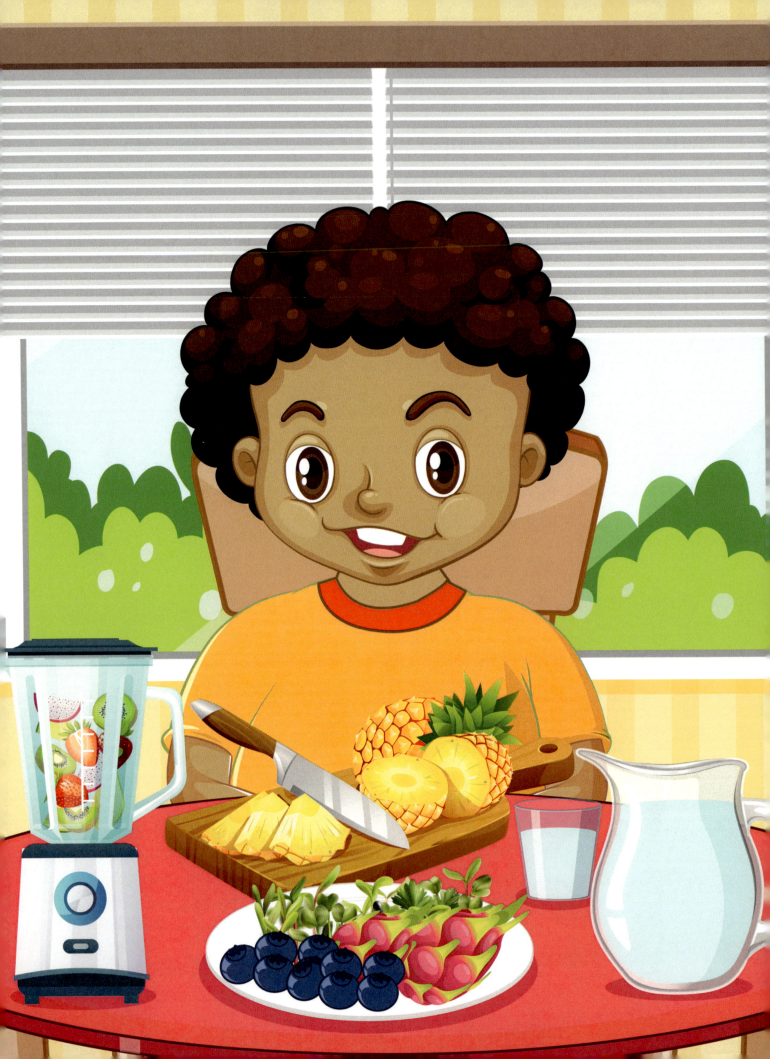

Philip was curious about Pineapples. They have a rough pattern on the outside. The best way to get the sweetness to the crown is to turn it upside down for a few days. The inside is bursting with bromelain. This enzyme makes it easier to break down proteins like meats you like to eat.

Philip takes chunks and makes a delicious smoothie. Of course, he adds water, dragon fruit, blueberries, and micro greens. Yum Yum.

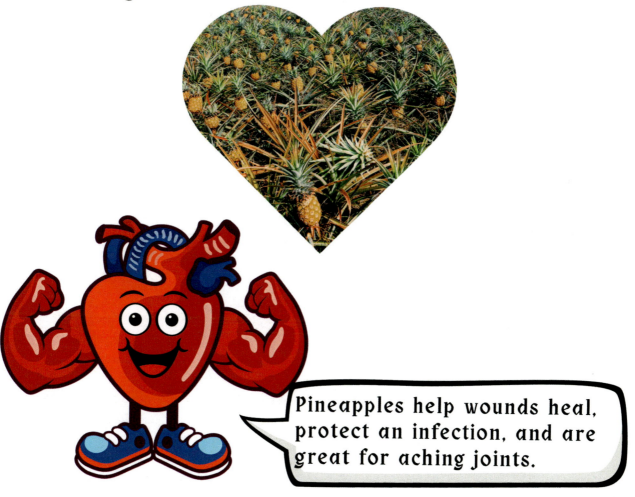

Pineapples help wounds heal, protect an infection, and are great for aching joints.

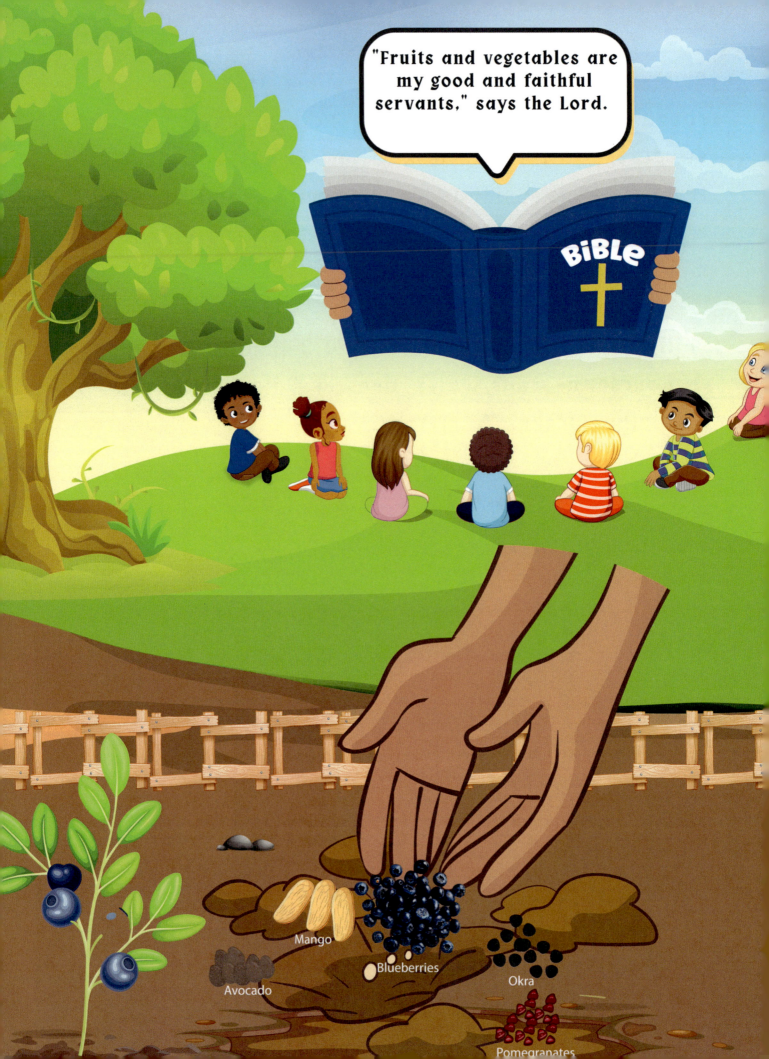

ABOUT the Author

Patricia K. Broadney is a retired Army Sergeant First Class. Currently, she works as a nutrition consultant. Patricia is married and has two children. In addition to her professional roles, she serves as a pastor and is a devoted servant of the Lord Jesus Christ.

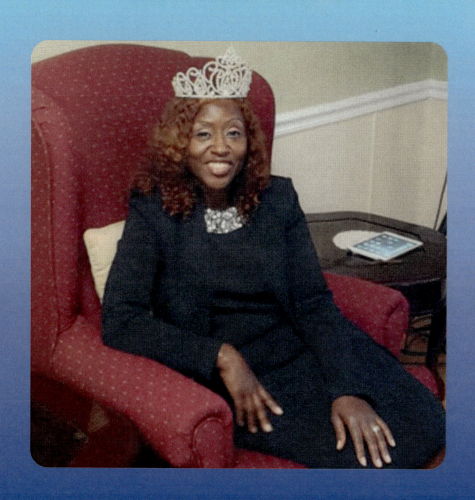

Made in the USA
Middletown, DE
14 January 2025